THE LUNGS

A Quick Guide to Lungs Health and Diseases

Joshua John

TABLE OF CONTENTS

INTRODUCTION

Welcome to the quick reference guide for the lungs!

Since we can only take in oxygen via our breath, the lungs, which are one of the most important organs in the body, are necessary for our continued existence.

The lungs are susceptible to a wide variety of illnesses and conditions, some of which are relatively harmless, like an infection of the respiratory system, while others are potentially lethal, such as lung cancer or chronic obstructive pulmonary disease (COPD).

Purpose of the Book

The purpose of this book is to act as a quick and easily accessible reference on the lungs, as well as the most prevalent lung ailments, their symptoms, diagnosis, and treatment options, as well as prevention measures.

The book is created for individuals who are interested in their lungs and want to learn more about how to keep them healthy. Additionally, the book is written for those who have been diagnosed with a lung condition and want to understand more about their sickness as well as various treatments.

Anatomy of the Lungs

The lungs are an essential component of the respiratory system of the body because they are responsible for exchanging carbon dioxide and oxygen with the air that surrounds a person.

The lungs are air sacs that are located inside the thoracic cavity of the chest, between the ribs for protection, and are divided into left and right lobes. The thoracic cavity is located between the sternum and the sternum.

Bronchioles are the smallest airways in the lung, and they surround each lobe of the lung like a network. Bronchioles encircle each lobe. Alveoli, which are very little air sacs, may be found at the very end of the bronchioles. They are the organelles that are in charge of gas exchange.

The pleura is a thin layer of tissue that surrounds the lungs and helps to protect and lubricate the lungs as they expand and contract with each breath. Its primary function is to keep the lungs from being damaged.

The diaphragm is a muscle that has the form of a dome and is located underneath the lungs. It regulates breathing by contracting and relaxing in order to change the size of the chest cavity as the body breathes in and out.

Function of the Lungs

The lungs are responsible for two primary functions: taking in oxygen and releasing carbon dioxide into the atmosphere.

When we breathe in, air travels from the nasal cavity through the trachea and bronchi to the smaller bronchioles and alveoli. It is in these areas that oxygen and carbon dioxide are expelled and taken in, respectively.

The oxygen that we breathe in via our lungs is then transported throughout the body by red blood cells and put to use in the production of energy in every cell.

At the same time, the carbon dioxide that is produced by our cells is transported back to the lungs by circulation. Once there, it is released into the alveoli, and it is then expelled from the body.

The lungs are responsible for more than simply the exchange of gasses; they also maintain the pH balance of the blood by regulating the amount of carbon dioxide that it contains.

The lungs work in conjunction with the immune system to protect the body against harmful infections and other chemicals that come from the outside.

CHAPTER I

COMMON LUNG CONDITIONS

There are many different lung conditions that can affect people of all ages and backgrounds. Here are some of the most common lung conditions:

Asthma

Asthma is a respiratory condition that restricts airflow across the airways and is characterized by persistent inflammation and narrowing of the bronchial tubes. This constriction may not only make it difficult to take in air, but it may also induce symptoms such as asthma, coughing, chest tightness, and shortness of breath.

Exertion, exposure to cold air, stress, or any variety of allergens or irritants are just some of the things that might bring on asthma symptoms. The severity and frequency of an asthmatic person's symptoms may vary anywhere from mild to severe to continual, and everything in between.

To accomplish the intended benefits of reducing inflammation and expanding airways during asthma therapy, it is sometimes necessary to take more than one medicine at a time.

This is the case with inhaled bronchodilators and corticosteroids, for example. Alterations to one's way of life, such as staying away from things that might set off an asthma attack and maintaining a high standard of respiratory cleanliness, may also help manage the condition.

Immunotherapy, also known as allergy injections, may be recommended for certain individuals who suffer from asthma to desensitize their immune systems to the triggers of their condition, which, in turn, results in a progressive lessening in the severity of their symptoms.

Chronic Obstructive Pulmonary Disease (COPD)

A defining characteristic of chronic obstructive pulmonary disease is a slow but steady loss of lung function over time (COPD). In most cases, a history of smoking or exposure to other irritants is associated with chronic obstructive pulmonary disease (COPD). COPD is an umbrella term for a range of respiratory illnesses, such as emphysema and chronic bronchitis.

Symptoms of COPD include but are not limited to the following: coughing, wheezing, chest tightness, and shortness of breath. As the patient's condition worsens, they run the risk of developing complications such as respiratory failure, pneumonia, and heart disease.

Although COPD cannot be cured, the symptoms may be treated and its progression can be delayed with the use of medicines. Inhaled bronchodilators and steroids, amongst other medications, are often used to treat

COPD. These treatments work by lowering inflammation and increasing airway diameter, respectively.

People who suffer from the chronic obstructive pulmonary disease (COPD) may find that participating in pulmonary rehabilitation, a program that improves lung function and quality of life via the use of physical activity, breathing techniques, and education, is beneficial to their condition. Treatment options for more severe cases may include oxygen therapy as well as surgical intervention.

Stopping smoking and avoiding exposure to other irritants, such as those found in the environment (such as air pollution) or the workplace (such as chemicals), is a key component in managing COPD and reducing the risk of complications.

Lung Cancer

Lung cancer is a form of cancer that begins in the lungs and is characterized by the uncontrollable proliferation of abnormal cells. The principal cause of this disease, which is responsible for the deaths of more people each year than all other types of cancer combined, is prolonged and repeated contact with cigarette smoke as well as other environmental toxins.

A persistent cough, chest tightness, shortness of breath, coughing up blood, and a loss of appetite that does not make sense are common signs and symptoms of lung cancer. However, the signs and symptoms of lung cancer may vary quite a little from patient to patient.

The stage of the illness and the patient's overall health are the two primary factors that define the degree to which lung cancer may be treated. One or more of the following modalities of treatment may be considered for a patient: surgery, chemotherapy, radiation therapy, or a combination of two or more of these treatments.

Immunotherapies and targeted therapies are the terms used to describe treatments that fight cancer cells by targeting specific genetic mutations or by stimulating the immune system to attack cancer cells.

Alterations in one's way of life, together with medical treatment, may help control the symptoms of lung cancer and lessen its severity. Quitting smoking and reducing your exposure to many other environmental toxins are two of the most important steps you can take to improve your lung cancer prognosis and reduce the likelihood that the disease will return.

Supportive care may take many forms, but some examples include nutritional counseling and palliative care, both of which have the potential to assist patients in coping with lung cancer symptoms and improve their quality of life overall. Early detection of lung cancer, achieved by screening technologies such as low-dose CT scans, may be beneficial to those who are at a high risk of developing the disease.

Pneumonia

Pneumonia is a contagious illness of the respiratory system that causes inflammation and fluid buildup in the lungs. Pneumonia may be caused by a large variety of different organisms in the microbiome.

A persistent cough, tightness in the chest, shortness of breath, fever, and chills are some of the most typical symptoms of pneumonia. The symptoms of pneumonia may appear in a broad variety of ways, depending on the underlying cause of the disease. In its most severe forms, pneumonia is capable of causing a wide range of major health complications, including sepsis, respiratory failure, and even death.

The most common therapy for bacterial pneumonia is the use of antibiotics or other medications that attack viruses or fungi rather than bacteria. In addition, over-the-counter (OTC) medications, such as cough suppressants and fever reducers, are available to aid in the treatment of symptoms.

Hospitalization is often recommended as the safest and most effective course of action if there is a need for life-sustaining interventions such as oxygen therapy or assisted mechanical respiration.

In conjunction with vaccines against many bacterial and viral infections, maintaining good respiratory hygiene is a key component of treating pneumonia. This includes practices such as washing one's hands often and avoiding proximity to others who are ill.

Taking precautions to avoid coming into contact with germs that might cause pneumonia is especially important for those who have immune systems that are already impaired or who suffer from underlying conditions such as chronic lung disease or heart disease.

Tuberculosis

The lung is the most prevalent location where Tuberculosis (TB), a bacterial illness that may spread to other parts of the body, is acquired. TB is the leading cause of death worldwide. Mycobacterium tuberculosis, the bacteria that causes tuberculosis (TB), may spread through the air and infect other people when an infected person coughs, sneezes, or even just speaks.

Several symptoms might point to TB, including a persistent cough, a high fever, nighttime sweats, and a lack of appetite. In some persons, the disease TB may not manifest any visible symptoms at all. *Do you have tuberculosis, either latent or active?*

A person is considered to have latent tuberculosis if they have the tuberculosis germs inside their body but the bacteria stay dormant and the person does not spread the disease to others. When TB is diagnosed as active, it means that the bacteria responsible for the disease are now doing their job and causing symptoms.

Patients with TB need to take a multitude of medications over many months for the treatment to be successful. It is essential to finish the prescribed course of treatment for the medication to eliminate the infection and reduce the risk of developing drug-resistant strains of tuberculosis.

An inpatient stay in a medical facility may provide round-the-clock monitoring and supportive care, as well as the assurance that all medications will be given in the correct dosages.

There are a variety of possible preventive strategies, including vaccination, the maintenance of high standards of respiratory hygiene, and the identification and treatment of those who are currently afflicted with an active case of tuberculosis.

Persons who work in healthcare, those who are in close contact with people who have active tuberculosis, and those who have immune systems that are not functioning properly all have an elevated risk of catching the illness and should be tested and monitored for tuberculosis infection.

CHAPTER II

SIGNS AND SYMPTOMS OF LUNG CONDITIONS

Shortness of Breath

Dyspnea, or difficulty breathing, has numerous causes. The list could go on and on, but some examples include pulmonary and cardiovascular diseases, anxiety, and obesity.

Obstruction of the airways, lung inflammation or infection, or diminished lung function as a consequence of lung disease are all potential causes of respiratory shortness of breath. Breathlessness might be caused by several respiratory diseases and conditions, including asthma, COPD, and interstitial lung disease.

In cardiovascular illness, shortness of breath may result from many factors, including a decrease in oxygen-rich blood flow to the lungs and/or cardiac muscle weakness. Shortness of breath may be a sign of heart or circulatory system conditions such as heart failure, pulmonary embolism, or heart valve malfunction.

In addition to anxiety and panic attacks, additional reasons for shortness of breath include weakened lung function and a reduced tolerance for physical effort.

Depending on the cause, medication may be used to treat shortness of breath, such as bronchodilators or steroids for respiratory disorders or diuretics and blood thinners for cardiovascular illnesses.

Depending on the severity of the patient's condition, doctors may recommend oxygen therapy and pulmonary rehabilitation. People who suffer from anxiety-related shortness of breath may find relief via stress management techniques including deep breathing exercises and meditation.

Treating the underlying cause of shortness of breath is the most effective method to avoid more episodes. This may include addressing a health issue that has been present for some time or making adjustments to one's lifestyle, such as becoming less overweight or giving up smoking. Regular exercise and good respiratory hygiene may help protect lung function and reduce the risk of respiratory infections.

Wheezing

Wheezing is the name given to the high-pitched whistling sound that occurs when air is driven into airways that have become limited or clogged. It is a symptom that may be brought on by a variety of diseases and conditions, including those that impact the respiratory system, allergies, and bronchospasm, amongst others.

Wheezing is a frequent symptom of respiratory illnesses and may be an indicator of airway inflammation or constriction, both of which may make it difficult to breathe. Wheezing can also be an indication of asthma.

The symptoms of wheezing may be triggered by some respiratory conditions, including asthma, chronic obstructive pulmonary disease (COPD), and bronchiolitis, among others.

In allergic illnesses such as allergic rhinitis and food allergies, a constriction of the airways and an inflammatory response may both contribute to wheezing.

Bronchospasm, which is the sudden contraction of the muscles around the airways, may also cause wheezing. Bronchospasm may be brought on by a wide variety of factors, some of the most common of which are physical activity, exposure to cold air, and allergies.

It is possible to treat wheezing using medications that reduce inflammation and relax the airways, such as bronchodilators and steroids; however, the therapy must be customized to the particular cause of the illness.

Oxygen therapy and other treatments that concentrate on the respiratory system could be recommended in certain cases. If you have allergies, you may reduce or eliminate the wheezing symptoms you experience by avoiding the allergens that set off your allergic reactions and using antihistamines or other allergy medications.

Making changes to one's lifestyle, such as avoiding known irritants or triggers, participating in regular exercise, and practicing basic respiratory hygiene, are a few of the many factors that may help prevent wheezing. With the aid of medical therapy, wheezing may be prevented. This is particularly true if the underlying condition, such as asthma or COPD, is under control.

Chest Pain

Anxiety and discomfort in the chest may be a sign of some different medical issues, such as those affecting the heart, lungs, digestive system, or musculoskeletal system.

It's very uncommon for chest pain to be accompanied by additional symptoms like shortness of breath, nausea, and sweating, although the pain itself might be either modest or severe.

Conditions affecting the heart, such as angina or a heart attack, may induce chest discomfort by cutting off the blood supply to the organ. Inflammation of the heart muscle (myocarditis) or the heart's lining (pericarditis) is another potential source of chest discomfort (pericarditis).

A collapsed lung, pneumonia, bronchitis, or any infection or inflammation of the lungs may all lead to chest discomfort (pneumothorax).

Chest discomfort may be brought on by a variety of different medical issues, including those affecting the digestive tract (such as acid reflux or gastritis) and the musculoskeletal system (such as costochondritis or a chest wall injury).

Medications like pain relievers and anti-inflammatory agents, as well as procedures like angioplasty and bypass surgery for cardiac issues, may be used to treat chest discomfort, but the treatment relies on determining the root cause.

It may be suggested that you make some changes to your way of life, such as cutting down on your weight or giving up cigarettes. People who have chest discomfort as a result of their worry may benefit from learning how to relax and de-stress via activities like deep breathing exercises or meditation.

Modifying your lifestyle with things like exercise and excellent respiratory hygiene, as well as treating any underlying medical concerns, might help prevent chest discomfort if you experience it. Keeping a good diet, not smoking, and not drinking excessively are all ways to lessen the likelihood of experiencing chest discomfort.

Coughing

Coughing is a reflexive action that helps clear the air passages of mucus, irritants, and foreign particles. Coughing helps clear the air passages since it is a reflex. It is a symptom that may manifest itself for a variety of distinct causes, including an infection in the respiratory system, allergies, asthma, or chronic obstructive pulmonary disease (COPD).

Coughing is a frequent symptom of respiratory infections such as the common cold and the flu. Coughing may be caused by inflammation or infection in the upper or lower respiratory tract. It's possible that the coughing that comes along with allergic disorders like hay fever and allergic rhinitis is caused by the immune system's inflammatory reaction to the condition.

Both asthma, a persistent condition that may cause coughing, and chronic obstructive pulmonary disease (COPD), a progressive lung disease that may cause coughing, wheezing, and shortness of breath, have their origins in airway inflammation and constriction. Asthma is a chronic disorder, and COPD is a progressive lung disease.

Coughing may also be triggered by the intake of irritants such as smoke or air pollution, or by the use of medications such as Angiotensin-Converting Enzyme (ACE) inhibitors. Both of these factors can be found in the environment.

A cough may be treated with a wide variety of medications and therapies, ranging from bronchodilators and steroids to oxygen therapy and pulmonary rehabilitation. These treatments are all taken in response to the underlying cause of the cough.

Those who suffer from allergies may be able to reduce their coughing by avoiding their allergens' triggers as well as utilizing antihistamines and other allergy medications.

Making modifications to one's lifestyle, such as avoiding known irritants or triggers, participating in regular exercise, and practicing good respiratory hygiene, are some of how one might prevent coughing.

Other methods include The treatment of any underlying medical conditions, such as asthma or COPD, which may result in a reduction in coughing.

Fatigue

The condition known as "fatigue" refers to a state of mental, emotional, or physical exhaustion that may be brought on by a wide variety of various stimuli. The severity of the condition may range from mild to severe, and it can either be acute or chronic.

Anemia, difficulties with the thyroid, persistent discomfort, and viruses like the flu or mononucleosis are all potential contributors to a person's experience of exhaustion.

A great number of conditions that last for a long time often manifest themselves with fatigue.

Exhaustion, which may be the consequence of a chemical imbalance in the brain or a chronic stress response, is a contributing factor in the development of depression and anxiety, which are both emotional and psychological diseases.

Several factors might play a role in one's day-to-day life that can lead to fatigue, including a lack of sleep, physical activity, or a healthy diet.

It's possible that making certain changes to one's lifestyle, including getting more sleep, working out more often, and improving one's diet, might be part of a successful treatment plan for fatigue.

Medication, such as antidepressants or stimulants, may also be advised; however, the underlying reason may influence this recommendation.

It is possible that altering one's lifestyle to include more rest, less stress, and abstinence from drug usage might prevent weariness, although this depends on the cause.

Keeping up with a consistent routine of physical activity and healthy food may help you avoid being worn out.

CHAPTER III

DIAGNOSIS AND TREATMENT OF LUNG CONDITIONS

Diagnostic Tests

Several diagnostic procedures exist for determining the cause of respiratory symptoms and assessing lung health. Standardized exams include:

- **Spirometry:** This is a basic test that determines how much air a person can intake and exhale, as well as how rapidly they can exhale. Asthma and chronic obstructive pulmonary disease are two of the disorders that this test may detect (COPD).

- **Chest X-Ray:** This test generates a picture of the chest and may be used to diagnose problems including pneumonia, lung cancer, and emphysema.

- **Computed Tomography (CT) Scan:** This is a more comprehensive kind of X-ray that may offer additional information about the lungs and surrounding structures. This procedure is often used in the evaluation of lung nodules and the diagnosis of lung cancer.

- **Bronchoscopy:** This is a process in which a short, flexible tube with a camera is inserted into the airways to assess the lungs and, if required, obtain tissue samples.

- **Pulmonary Function Testing:** These tests assess how effectively the lungs perform and may assist in the diagnosis of illnesses such as interstitial lung disease.

- **Arterial Blood Gas Test:** This test monitors the levels of oxygen and carbon dioxide in the blood and may aid in the diagnosis of illnesses including chronic obstructive pulmonary disease (COPD) and asthma.

- **Sputum Culture:** This test includes studying a sample of mucus from the lungs to detect any bacteria or other organisms that may be causing respiratory symptoms.

The patient's symptoms, medical history, and the results of the physical examination will all play a role in determining which diagnostic test(s) to prescribe.

Medications

Medical intervention for the respiratory system and the lungs may be achieved via a wide variety of pharmaceutical options. The diagnosis and treatment plan will determine which medicine or combination of medications will be prescribed.

These are some of the most often prescribed drugs for treating respiratory disorders:

- **Bronchodilators:** These drugs relax the muscles in the airways, making it easier to breathe. Asthma and chronic obstructive pulmonary disease are only two of the many illnesses that these drugs are used to treat (COPD). Inhalers such as albuterol, salmeterol, and tiotropium are all examples of bronchodilators.

- **Inhaled corticosteroids:** These drugs are used to treat illnesses such as asthma by reducing inflammation in the airways. Fluticasone, budesonide, and mometasone are examples of corticosteroids that may be breathed.

- **Antihistamines:** These drugs prevent histamine, a substance generated during an allergic response, from acting. To alleviate symptoms of allergies and related disorders including allergic rhinitis, they are often prescribed. Some common antihistamines are loratadine, cetirizine, and fexofenadine.

- **Leukotriene Modifiers:** These drugs work by blocking the effects of leukotrienes, which are substances that may induce inflammation in the airways. Asthma and other breathing disorders are common uses. Drugs like montelukast and zafirlukast are leukotriene modifiers.

- **Antibiotics:** These drugs are used to treat bacterial illnesses such as pneumonia. Amoxicillin, azithromycin, and levofloxacin are only a few examples of antibiotics.

- **Chemotherapy:** Chemotherapy is a treatment option for several forms of cancer, including lung cancer. Cancer cells, and other rapidly proliferating cells, are the primary targets of chemotherapy drugs.

- **Immunotherapy:** Immunotherapy is a relatively recent kind of medical treatment that is used in the management of some kinds of lung cancer. To fight cancer, immunotherapy boosts the immune system so that it can destroy diseased tissue.

To find the right drug (or combination of medications) for your health issue, it's best to consult with a medical professional. They can help you figure out what to take and how much, how to avoid unwanted effects, and how to pair medications safely.

Lifestyle Changes

The chance of developing respiratory problems may be reduced, and lung health can be enhanced, by adopting a few simple lifestyle adjustments. Some adjustments in habits that are good for the lungs are as follows:

- **Quit Smoking:** Smoking is a substantial risk factor for lung cancer, chronic obstructive pulmonary disease (COPD), and other respiratory disorders. You may do a lot for your lungs just by giving up smoking.

- **Avoid Being Exposed to Air Pollution:** Air pollution may irritate the lungs and aggravate illnesses like asthma. Fire smoke, industrial pollutants, and other forms of air pollution should be avoided at all costs.

- **Exercise Regularly:** Participating in regular physical activity has been shown to enhance lung function and decrease the chance of developing respiratory diseases. Try to get at least 30 minutes of moderate activity, such as brisk walking, most days of the week.

- **Learn to Practice Personal Hygiene:** The symptoms of colds and the flu may be made much more uncomfortable if you don't take the time to maintain excellent hygiene and wash your hands often.

- **Maintain a Healthy Weight:** Being overweight may put additional pressure on the lungs and raise the risk of respiratory illnesses. Achieve a healthy weight by adhering to a nutrition plan and getting enough exercise.

- **Manage Stress:** Because stress may aggravate respiratory problems, finding techniques to manage stress is critical. Meditation, yoga, and deep breathing exercises are all examples of methods that might help you unwind.

- **Avoid Allergens:** If you have allergies, try to avoid allergens that make your symptoms worse. Some examples include pollen, dust mites, and animal dander.

Protect your lungs and lower your chance of developing respiratory problems by adopting these habits. It is essential, however, that you consult your doctor to figure out the best course of action.

Surgery

Certain lung disorders may need surgical intervention to be treated effectively.

The following are some of the most frequent procedures involving the lungs:

- **Lobectomy:** A lobectomy is a surgical procedure in which a section of the lung is surgically removed. Lung cancer and other diseases that only affect one lung lobe can need this procedure.

- **Pneumonectomy:** This is a form of surgery in which the whole lung is removed. When treating lung cancer or other diseases that involve the whole lung, this procedure may be required.

- **Wedge Resection:** This is a form of surgery in which a little wedge-shaped portion of lung tissue is excised. Possible medical uses include making a diagnosis or administering treatment.

- **Video-Assisted Thoracoscopic Surgery (VATS):** This is a form of minimally invasive surgery that involves inserting a tiny camera and surgical equipment into the chest via small incisions. In certain cases, such as lung cancer or pneumothorax, it may be utilized as a diagnostic tool or therapeutic intervention (collapsed lung).

- **Open Thoracotomy:** This is a more intrusive form of surgery that involves making a wide incision in the chest. More extensive treatment plans or bigger tissue samples may need this.

When deciding whether surgery is the right course of treatment for you, your doctor will weigh the potential advantages and drawbacks of the operation. Pre and post-operative care, such as pain management, breathing exercises, and rehabilitation, may also be discussed.

Palliative Care

Palliative care is a subcategory of medical therapy that emphasizes comfort and the relief of pain for patients who are diagnosed with a terminal illness.

The patient and their loved ones get support on an emotional and spiritual level, in addition to assistance with their physical symptoms, which may include pain, shortness of breath, and fatigue.

Palliative treatment may be of value to patients who are in the latter stages of lung cancer or other serious lung disorders. This is particularly true if the patients are having difficulty keeping their symptoms under control.

Palliative care doesn't try to treat the root cause of the patient's pain. Instead, it focuses on easing the patient's symptoms and improving their quality of life.

Palliative care may require the participation of a large number of different members of a healthcare team, including but not limited to physicians, nurses, social workers, and chaplains.

Their collaboration yields a treatment plan that is singularly adapted to the patient's condition, personal preferences, and intended objectives, and it is as a direct consequence of their combined efforts that this plan is developed.

Palliative care may be administered in a variety of settings, including hospitals, hospice facilities, and even the patient's own home, if necessary. In addition to conventional medical treatment, such as chemotherapy or radiation therapy, it can be given to the patient as an option.

If you or a member of your family is struggling with a terminal lung condition, you should talk to your physician about the possibility of receiving palliative treatment.

They are in a better position to describe the resources that are available to you and advise you on whether or not palliative care is a suitable match for your circumstances than you are. You are in the best position to explain the resources that are available to you.

CHAPTER IV

MAINTAINING LUNG HEALTH

Giving up on Smoking

One of the most effective ways for people to improve their lung health is to quit smoking. Quitting smoking might lessen one's chances of acquiring lung cancer, chronic obstructive pulmonary disease, or any of the other many lung ailments that smoking causes.

If you want to stop smoking, consider these suggestions.

- **Prepare Ahead of Time:** Determine when you will stop smoking and how you will handle the urges and withdrawal. To alleviate distress, you may want to try nicotine replacement therapy or other drugs.

- **Learn How to Get Help:** Share your decision to stop smoking with loved ones and solicit their encouragement as you make the transition. You may want to see a therapist or other medical professional or join a support group.

- **Locate Your Smoking Triggers:** Think about what causes you to reach for a cigarette and figure out how to deal with those circumstances without resorting to smoking. Rather than lighting up after eating, consider taking a stroll.

- **Be Productive:** keep your body and mind active by engaging in physical and mental pursuits.

- **Avoid Those Temptation:** Avoid circumstances or locations where you may be tempted to smoke, such as bars or parties.

- **Honor Your Little Achievements:** Whether you've gone a week or a month without lighting up, you should be proud of yourself.

It's important to keep in mind that quitting smoking is a procedure that may need more than one try. Don't give up if you have a lapse and smoke again. If anything, use this setback as motivation to redouble your efforts to finally kick the habit.

To safeguard one's lungs and one's entire health and well-being, quitting smoking is crucial but not easy.

Exercising Regularly

Working out regularly is crucial for maintaining healthy lungs. Exercising regularly may boost lung capacity, enhance stamina, and decrease the likelihood of developing lung disorders like COPD.

Here are some tips for making regular exercise part of your routine:

- **Begin Slowly:** If you're new to exercise or have been inactive for a long, begin with low-impact activities like walking, swimming, or cycling. Workouts should be built up in both length and intensity over time.

- **Select Fun Activities:** Physical activity has been shown to improve mood and quality of life, so pick something you like doing. For long-term success with your fitness plan, this is a crucial factor.

- **Integrate Strength Training:** In addition to cardiovascular activity, including strength training activities such as lifting weights or practicing bodyweight exercises. It's a great way to become stronger and fitter.

- **Maintain Consistency:** Try to get at least 30 minutes of moderate-intensity exercise most days of the week. To get the advantages of exercise for lung health, you must be consistent in your efforts.

- **Listen to Your Body:** If you suffer shortness of breath or other symptoms when exercising, slow down or take a break. If you have any concerns about exercising with a lung ailment, you should discuss them with your doctor.

Regular exercise is essential for optimal lung health, but anybody, especially those with preexisting lung conditions, should see their doctor before beginning a new exercise program. They can advise you on the most appropriate kind of exercise and its level of intensity given your specific situation.

Keeping Air Pollution At Bay

Due to the link between lung illness and exposure to air pollution, limiting one's exposure to such pollutants is crucial for lung health protection. To lessen the impact of air pollution, consider these measures:

- Check The Air Quality Index: Keep a watch on the air quality index in your region, which monitors the number of contaminants in the air. Do not go outside if the air quality is bad, or think about using a mask if you must.

- Minimize Your Exposure To Indoor Pollutants: Because indoor air may be contaminated, you should take precautions to limit your exposure to indoor pollutants such as smoking, mold, and dust. Avoid smoking and secondhand smoke exposure, keep your house clean and dry and use a HEPA air filter.

- Use Public Transportation Or Carpool: When feasible, reduce your contribution to air pollution by using public transit, carpooling, or walking or bicycling.

- Avoid Exercising Outside During High-Pollution Periods: Exercise is good for lung health, but it's recommended to avoid it when pollution is severe. Take your workout inside or at a time of day with less pollution if you can.

- Be Careful Of Outdoor Activities: When planning outdoor activities, try to choose areas and times of day that have lower pollution levels. In place of a trek beside a busy road, maybe you might visit a park instead.

To preserve one's lungs and lower one's chance of developing lung disease, people should take measures to limit their exposure to air pollution.

Having a Healthy Diet

The maintenance of healthy lungs is dependent on a balanced diet and lifestyle. Here are some ways to improve your diet and lifestyle to better support lung health:

- **Consume a Well-Rounded Diet:** Aim for a diet that is abundant in fruits, vegetables, whole grains, lean proteins, and healthy fats. These foods are rich in antioxidants, vitamins, and minerals that have been shown to benefit respiratory health.

- **Foods Having Anti-Inflammatory Qualities Should Be Consumed:** Since chronic inflammation may lead to lung disorders, pick anti-inflammatory foods such as leafy greens, almonds, and fatty salmon.

- **Stay Hydrated:** Drink lots of water and other fluids to help keep your airways moist and hydrated.

- **Avoid Processed Meals:** Processed foods are generally rich in chemicals and preservatives that may be damaging to lung health. Instead of eating processed meals, go for whole ones.

- **Limit Your Intake of Alcohol and Caffeine:** Excessive alcohol and caffeine consumption may dehydrate the body and make breathing harder for those who have lung issues. Try cutting down to moderate amounts.

- **Speak With a Healthcare Expert:** If you have a lung issue, consult with a healthcare practitioner or a certified dietitian for specialized dietary advice.

The health of your lungs and body as a whole may be improved by adopting a more nutritious diet. To keep your lungs healthy and avoid illnesses like asthma and COPD from developing, it is important to eat a diet rich in colorful, whole foods.

Vaccinations

Lung-affecting respiratory disorders are preventable in part via vaccinations. Common immunizations that defend lung health are as follows:

- **Influenza Vaccination:** The influenza vaccine, sometimes known as the flu shot, is recommended yearly for most people, especially those who are at high risk of flu complications, such as small children, the elderly, and persons with lung diseases.

- **Pneumococcal Vaccination:** The pneumococcal vaccine aids in the prevention of pneumococcal disease, a dangerous bacterial infection that may cause pneumonia, meningitis, and other disorders.

- **COVID-19 Vaccine:** The COVID-19 vaccination protects against the SARS-CoV-2 virus's respiratory disease. All healthy adults over the age of 12 should have the vaccination, but those who are at high risk for COVID-19 problems should get it even sooner.

- **TDAP Vaccination:** The Tdap vaccine protects against tetanus, diphtheria, and pertussis (whooping cough), all of which may cause respiratory issues and catastrophic consequences.

- **Varicella Vaccination:** The varicella vaccine protects against chickenpox, which may be dangerous in certain people, especially those with compromised immune systems.

Individuals may help protect themselves and others from respiratory infections that can harm lung health by following the immunization protocols that are advised.

Consult your doctor about the immunizations that are most appropriate for your age, health, and way of life.

CHAPTER V

CONCLUSION

In conclusion, the lungs play a crucial role in the respiratory system by allowing the body to take in oxygen and release carbon dioxide. Lungs are susceptible to many different diseases and disorders, from the more common asthma and pneumonia to the more life-threatening lung cancer and chronic obstructive pulmonary disease (COPD).

To preserve lung health and avoid more severe effects, early diagnosis and treatment of these disorders are essential. A robust and healthy set of lungs may be maintained in addition to medical therapy by adopting good lifestyle choices including not smoking, eating well, and exercising regularly. Getting competent medical counsel is essential if you are worried about your lung health.

A Review of Lung Disorders and their Treatments

The lungs, to review, are crucial because they allow us to take in oxygen and release it throughout our bodies. Asthma, chronic obstructive pulmonary disease (COPD), lung cancer, pneumonia, TB, and other lung-related illnesses are all too common.

Depending on the nature and severity of the problem, different lung disorders may need different treatments. Medications like bronchodilators, steroids, and antibiotics are often prescribed, but lifestyle adjustments like giving up smoking, getting regular exercise, staying away from air pollution, and eating healthily are also important. It may be required to resort to surgical intervention or palliative treatment in some situations.

Vaccinations, frequent checkups with a healthcare expert, and early diagnosis may all play a role in protecting against lung disorders and managing symptoms in addition to the therapies listed above.

If you have symptoms or worries regarding your lung health, you must see a medical practitioner. Many people with lung issues may recover from their illnesses and live normal, active lives with the help of medical professionals.

Preventative Measures Such as Early Diagnosis and Treatment are Crucial.

When it comes to lung disorders, early identification, and treatment are critical for improving outcomes and quality of life. Signs and symptoms of lung diseases such as lung cancer and Chronic Obstructive Pulmonary Disease (COPD) are sometimes vague or nonexistent in the first stages.

However, many problems may be detected before they worsen and become harder to cure if people have frequent checkups and screening tests.

The expenses of medical care and the number of people who end up in the hospital may be lowered by early diagnosis and treatment, and the results will be better, too. People may save money and time by taking care of their health early on rather than waiting until it becomes a more serious or advanced problem.

People with lung diseases might benefit from receiving therapy early to reduce their symptoms and increase their quality of life. Individuals may learn to manage their disease and maintain an active and healthy lifestyle by working closely with a healthcare provider and adhering to a treatment plan.

Overarchingly, better outcomes and quality of life for those with lung disorders may be achieved through early identification and treatment. If you have a family history of lung problems or other risk factors, you must see a doctor about the screening tests and checkups they prescribe for you.

Final Thoughts and Resources for Further Information.

Here are some things to think about and some places to go for further data.

To breathe and get oxygen, the lungs are essential organs. Various lung disorders may be diagnosed and treated successfully so that patients can resume normal, active lifestyles.

Communicating with a medical expert about any symptoms or concerns you may have about your lungs is essential. Screenings, checkups, and treatment plans may be suggested by your doctor to aid in disease management and recovery.

Individuals and their families dealing with lung diseases have access to a wealth of helpful information. Here are some places to look for further information:

- Lung.org is the official website of the *American Lung Association,* a non-profit organization dedicated to improving the quality of life for people of all ages who are affected by lung disease.

- If you want to learn more about lung health and illness, you may visit the *National Heart, Lung, and Blood Institute* (nhlbi.nih.gov), a federal agency.

- To learn more about how to avoid and effectively treat respiratory diseases, check out the *Centers for Disease Control and Prevention* (cdc.gov).

- For those who suffer from asthma and allergies, "aafa.org" is the official website for the *Asthma and Allergy Foundation of America*, it is a nonprofit group that offers support, advocacy, and education.

These options represent a small subset of the extensive library at your disposal. The best way to manage your lung ailment and enhance your quality of life is to engage with your healthcare provider and reliable resources.

HERE ARE THE MOST VITAL QUERIES AND THEIR ANSWERS

Lung Transplant for Cystic Fibrosis?

A Lung Transplant for Cystic Fibrosis (CF) is a significant operation in which healthy donor lungs replace the damaged ones. A lung transplant for people with cystic fibrosis may have life-changing effects, including prolonging their life expectancy and enhancing their quality of life. When a patient's health improves, their quality of life improves along with it. However, there are certain hazards associated with the treatment, and it is crucial to have ongoing care thereafter.

Lunger Meaning?

A person with a lung problem, often a chronic respiratory illness such as cystic fibrosis, asthma, or chronic obstructive pulmonary disease (COPD), is sometimes referred to as a "langer." To put it another way, it's a term for describing someone who has trouble breathing regularly.

How Big are the Lungs?

Lung capacity may change with age, sex, height, weight, and health. The lungs of an adult are typically 12-20 cm (5-8 in) in length and 10-12 cm (4-5 in) in breadth (4-5 inches). However, there is a wide range in lung sizes because of factors like genetics and lifestyle. Asthma and chronic obstructive pulmonary disease (COPD) are only two examples of diseases that may reduce lung capacity.

Carcinogen

An agent or substance with the capability of causing cancer is called a carcinogen. Cancer-causing agents may take the shape of chemicals, radiation, or even viruses. Mutations in cancer-causing genes may result from exposure to carcinogens, which can harm DNA and other genetic material. Cigarette smoke, asbestos, benzene, and UV radiation from the sun are all examples of carcinogens.

As far as possible, reducing your contact with known carcinogens is crucial for keeping cancer at bay.

Orthopnea

When a person has orthopnea, they have trouble breathing when resting flat. Those who suffer from orthopnea typically find that they can breathe easier when they sit up straight or prop themselves up with many cushions. In most cases, the presence of orthopnea indicates the presence of a more serious heart or lung ailment, such as congestive heart failure, COPD, or asthma. Orthopnea treatment often entails attending to both the underlying cause and the symptoms. You should visit a doctor right away if you're having trouble breathing or if you're showing any other worrying symptoms.

Better Lungs Walgreens

Walgreens' Better Lungs range of all-natural vitamins is designed to promote healthy breathing. It is hoped that using these items can aid with inflammation, respiratory health, and general lung function. Herbal extracts, essential oils, vitamins, and minerals make up the line's focus on pulmonary health.

www.ingramcontent.com/pod-product-compliance
Lightning Source LLC
Chambersburg PA
CBHW061617250726
48653CB00019B/2724